PACU Nurse
Journal/Notebook

nurse

{ners} n. a scrub wearing, smile bringing, life saving rockstar who lives to heal and loves to encourage.

See also: SUPERHERO

This book belongs to:

_____

DATE: _____

_____

_____

_____

_____

_____

_____

_____

_____

_____

_____

_____

_____

_____

_____

_____

_____

_____

_____

_____

_____

DATE: _____

DATE: _____

DATE: _____

DATE: _____

DATE: _____

DATE: _____

DATE: _____

DATE: _____

DATE: _____

DATE: _____

DATE: _____

DATE: _____

DATE: _____

DATE: _____

DATE: _____

DATE: _____

DATE: _____

DATE: _____

DATE: _____

DATE: _____

DATE: _____

DATE: _____

DATE: _____

DATE: _____

DATE: _____

DATE: _____

DATE: _____

DATE: _____

DATE: _____

DATE: _____

DATE: _____

DATE: _____

DATE: _____

DATE: _____

DATE: _____

DATE: _____

DATE: _____

DATE: _____

DATE: _____

DATE: _____

DATE: _____

DATE: _____

DATE: _____

DATE: _____

DATE: _____

DATE: _____

DATE: _____

DATE: _____

DATE: _____

DATE: _____

DATE: _____

DATE: _____

DATE: _____

DATE: _____

Quotes from Patients

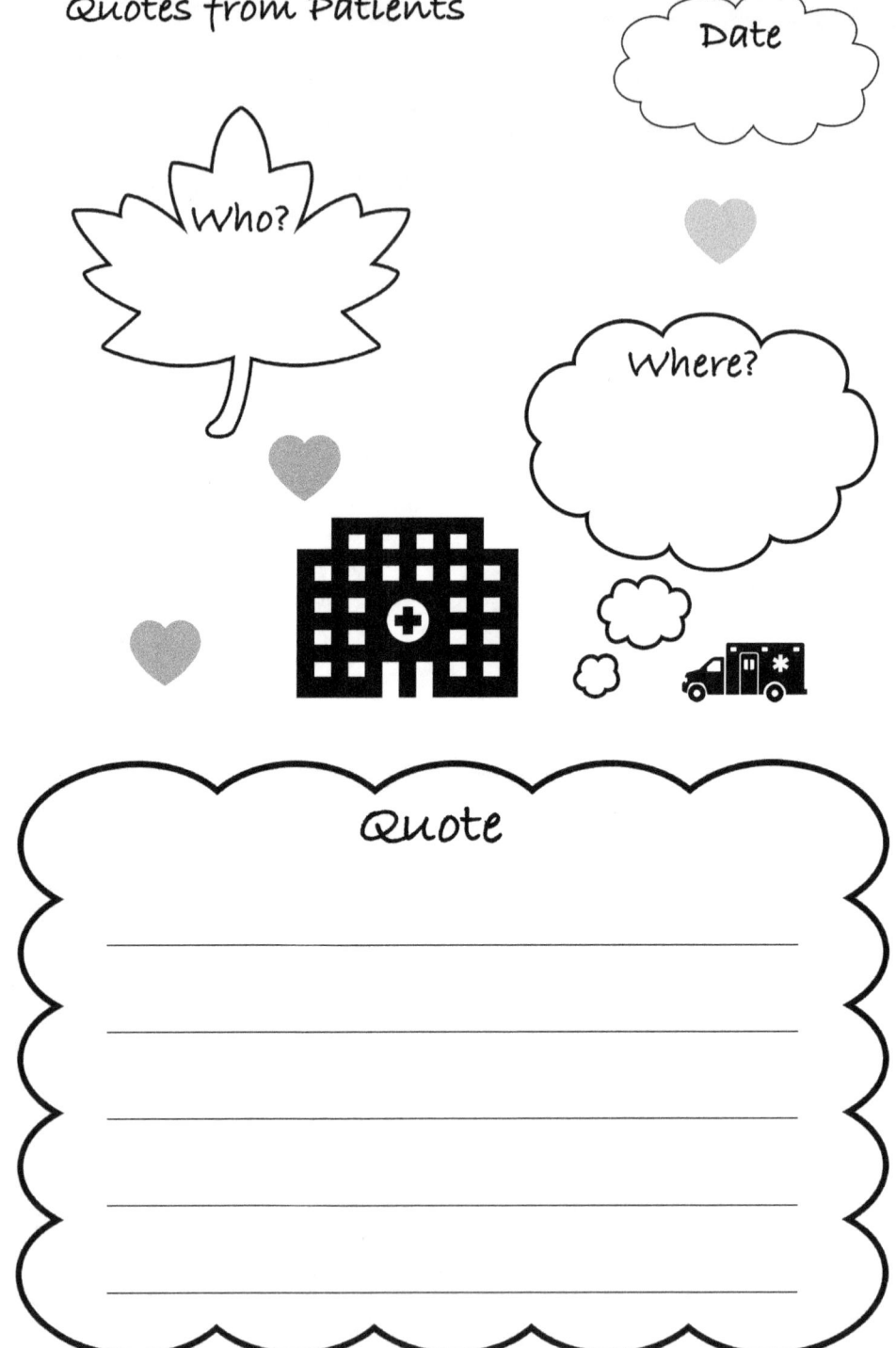

Date

Who?

Where?

Quote

_____
_____
_____
_____
_____

Quotes from Patients

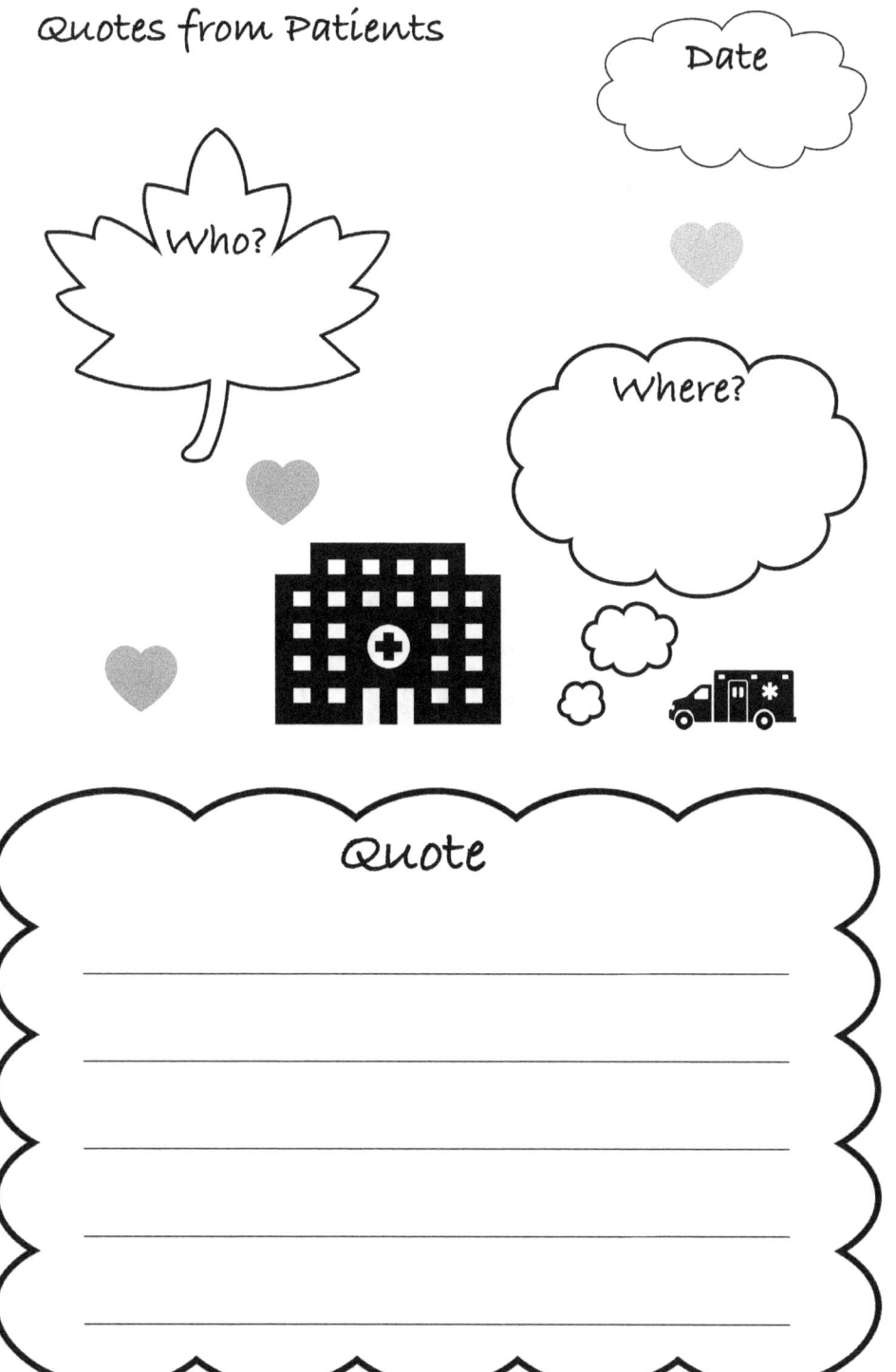

Date

Who?

Where?

Quote

Quotes from Patients

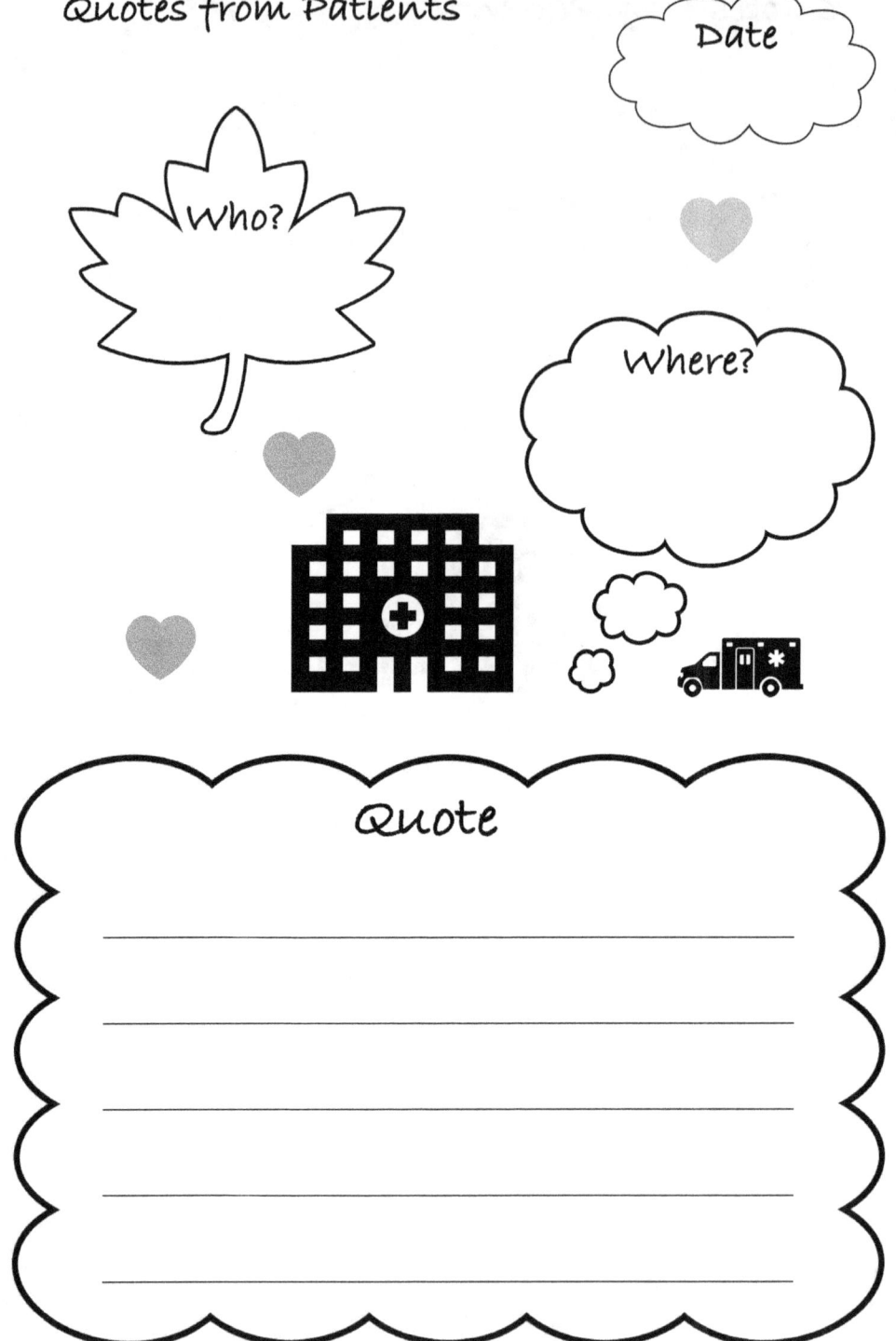

Date

Who?

Where?

Quote

Quotes from Patients

Date

Who?

Where?

Quote

_____

_____

_____

_____

_____

_____

Quotes from Patients

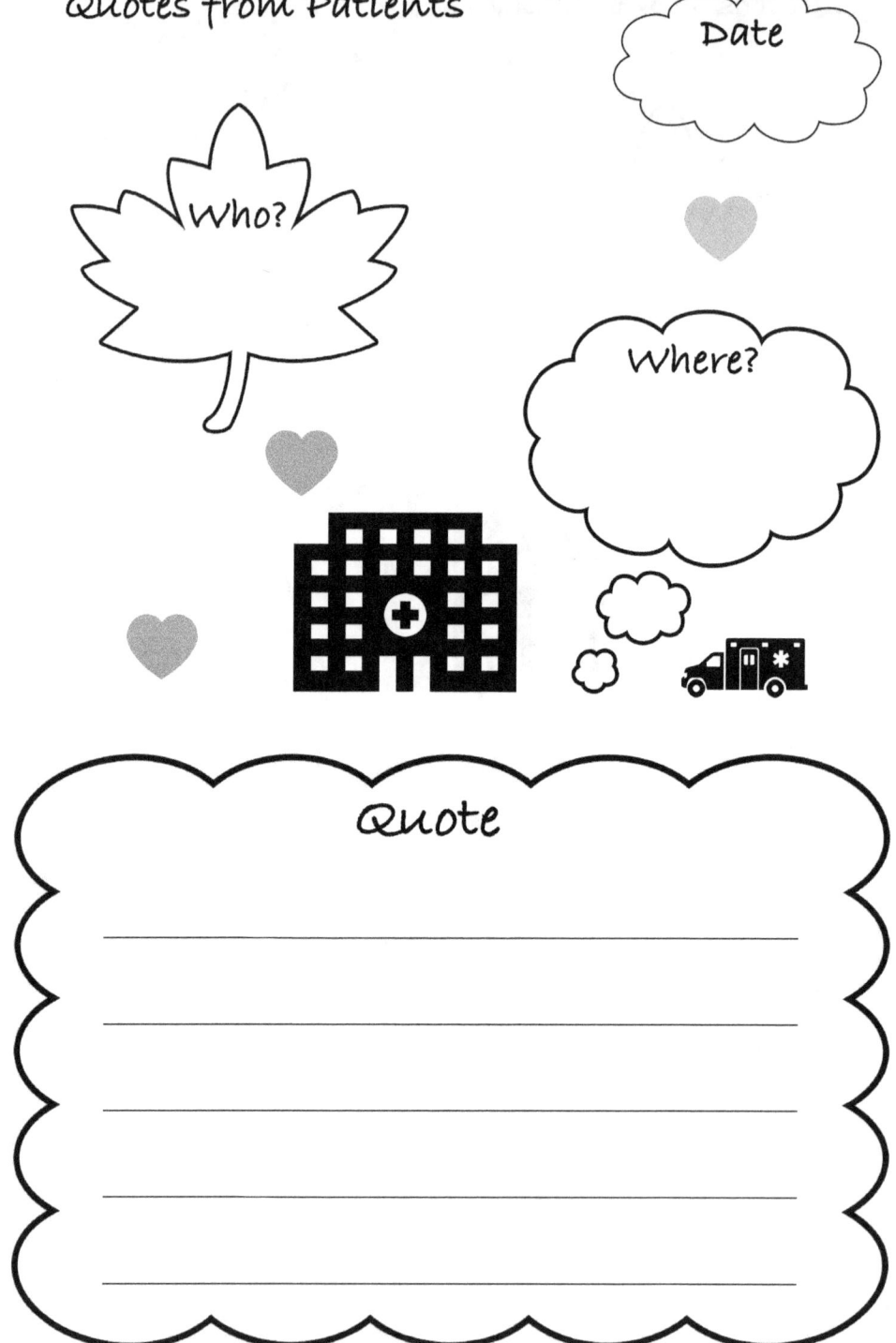

Date

Who?

Where?

Quote

Coloring Section

I Had Fun Once, Then
I Went To Nursing School

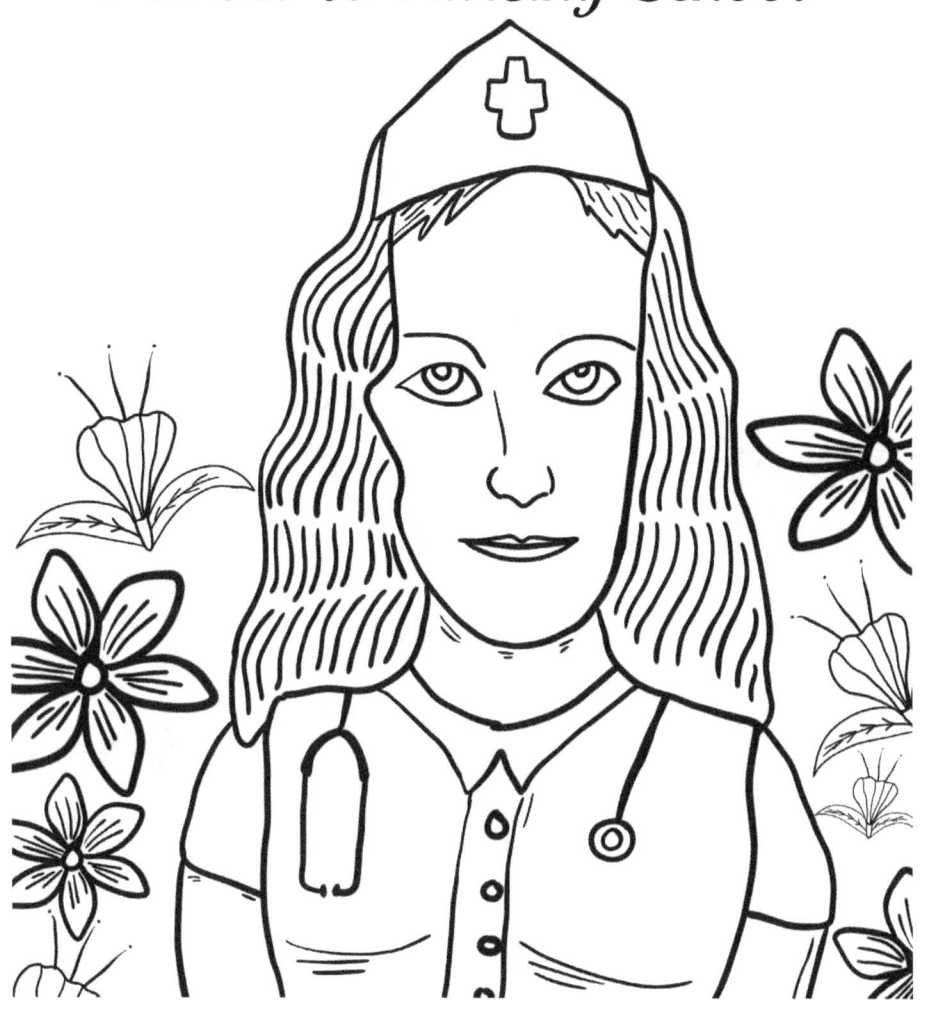

Ativan A Nurse's Best Friend

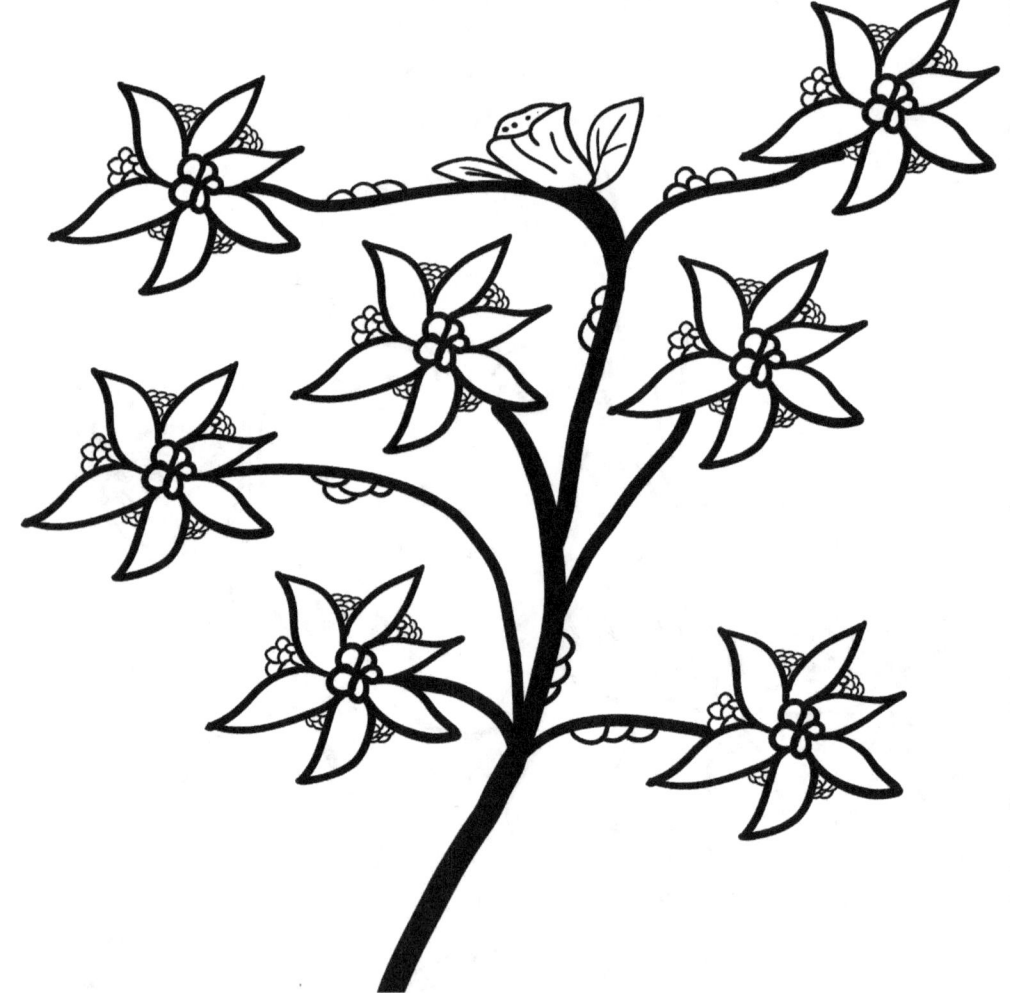

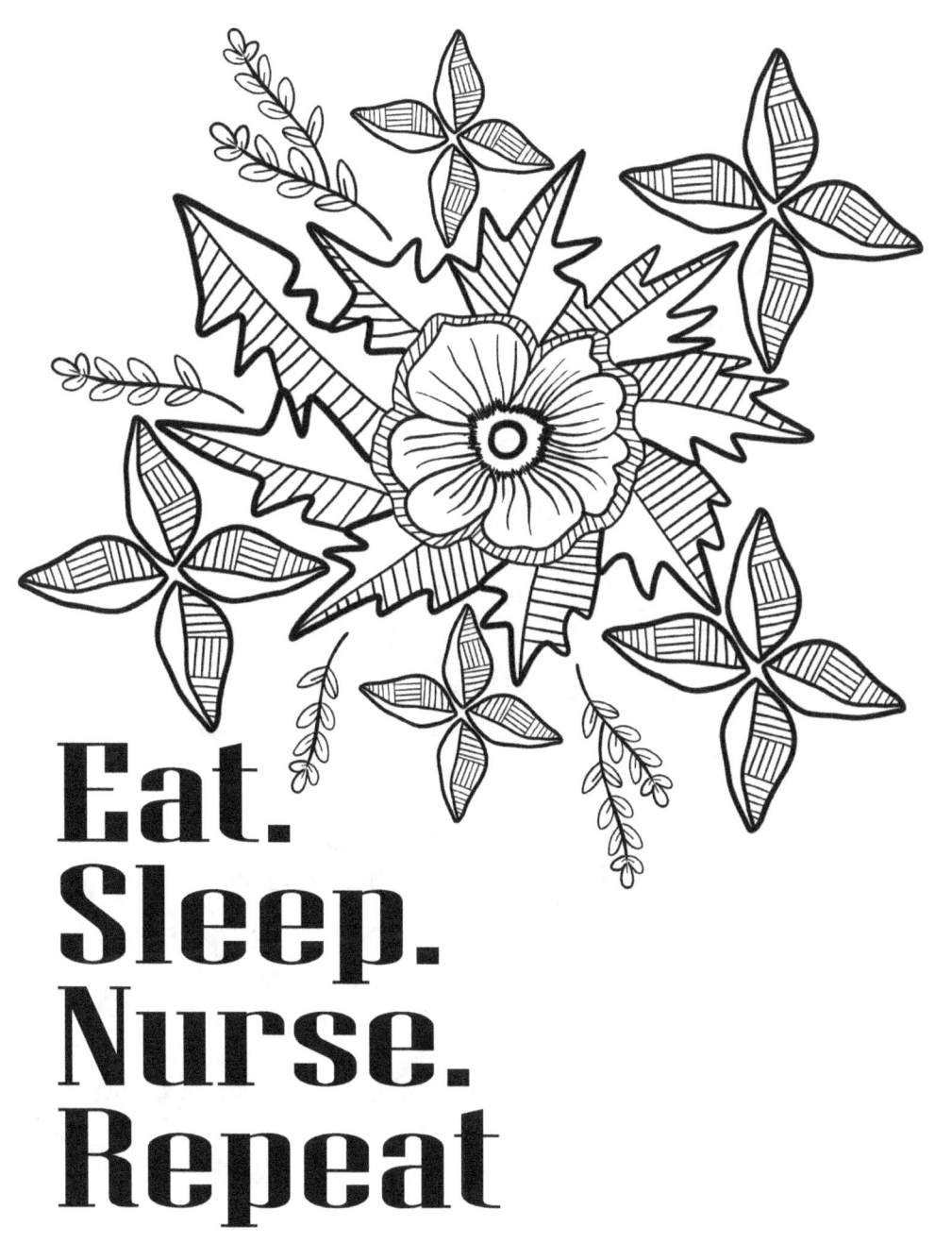

Eat.
Sleep.
Nurse.
Repeat

DO NOT MAKE ME SEDATE YOU.

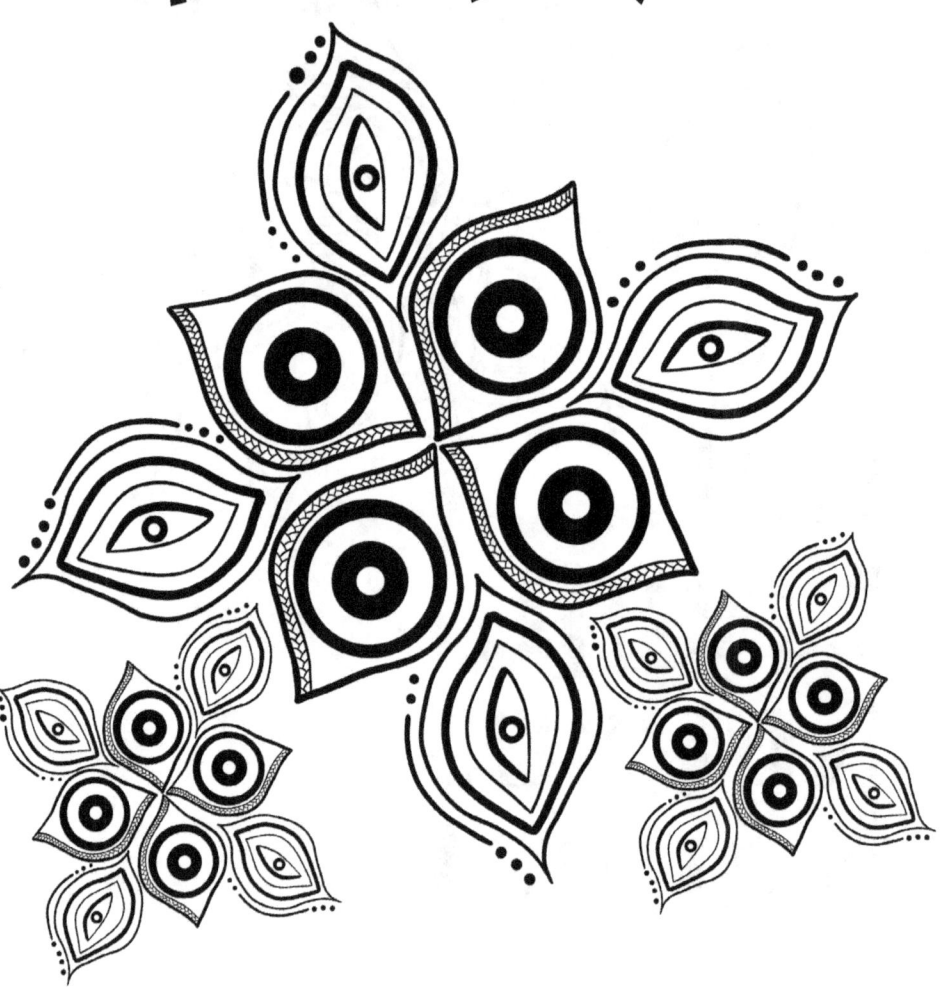

Best Nurse Ever

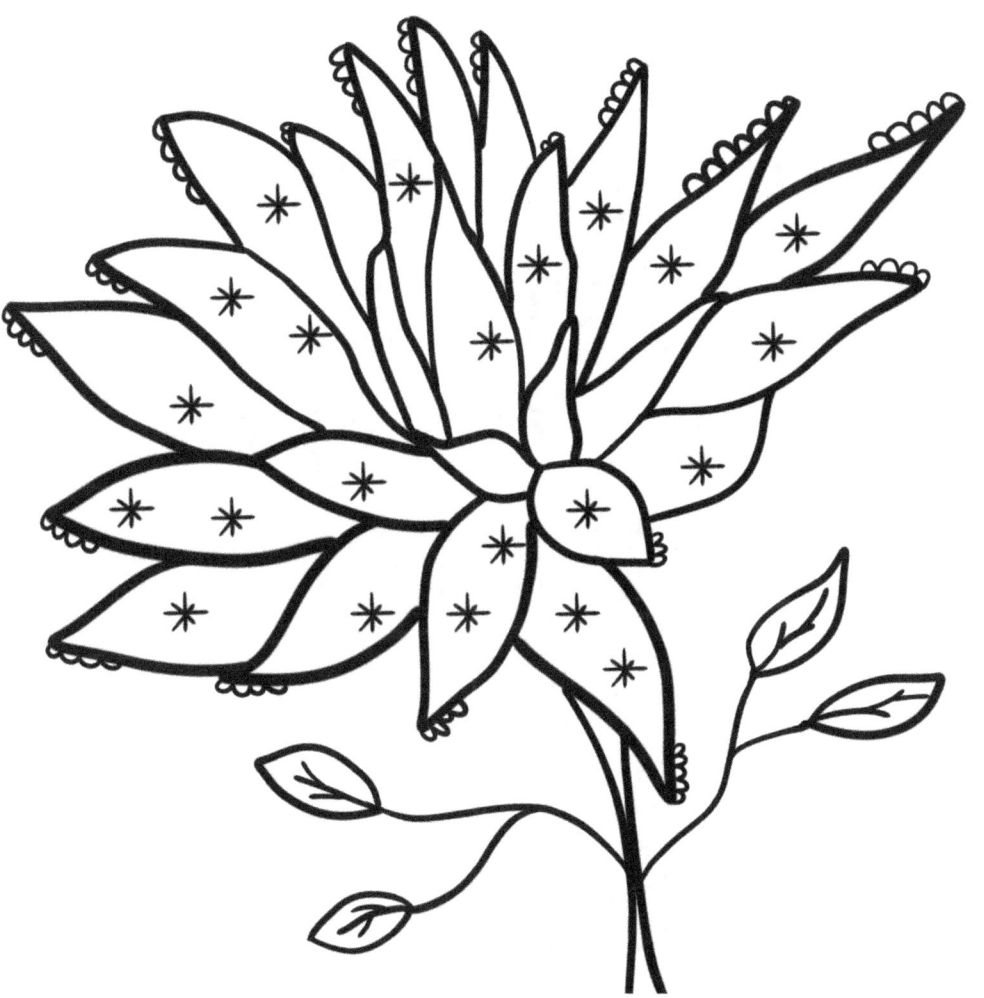

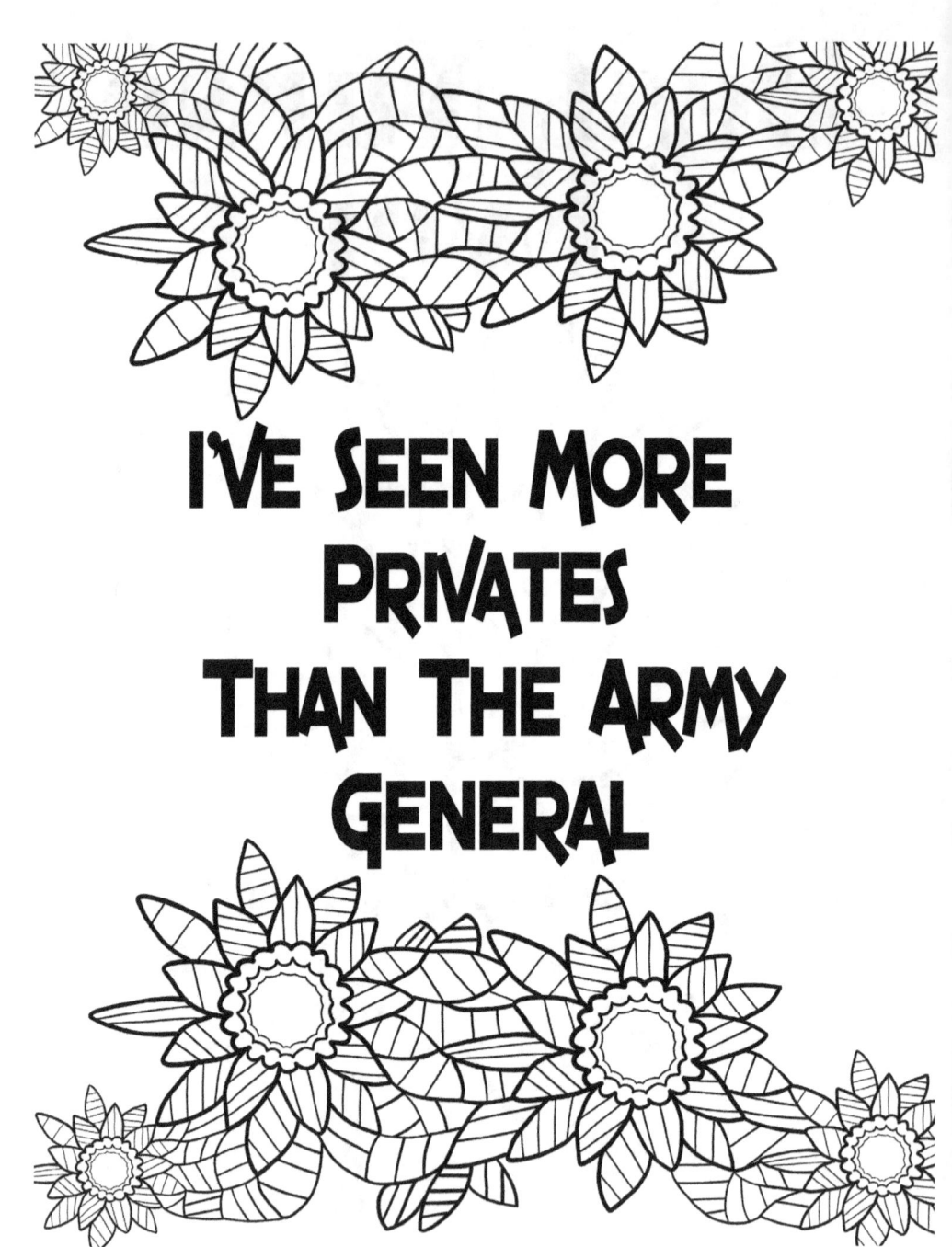

I'VE SEEN MORE
PRIVATES
THAN THE ARMY
GENERAL

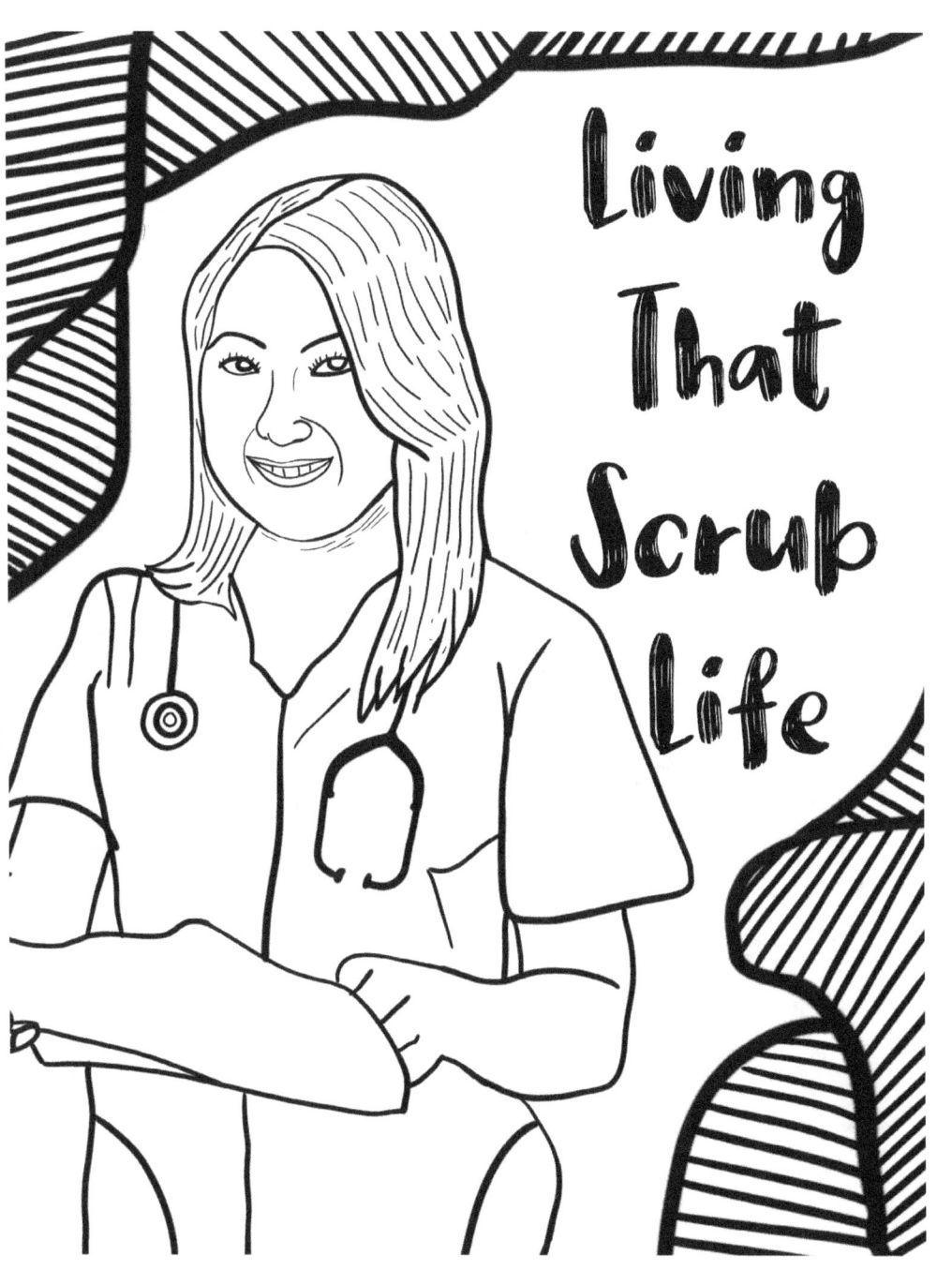

Nurse Squad

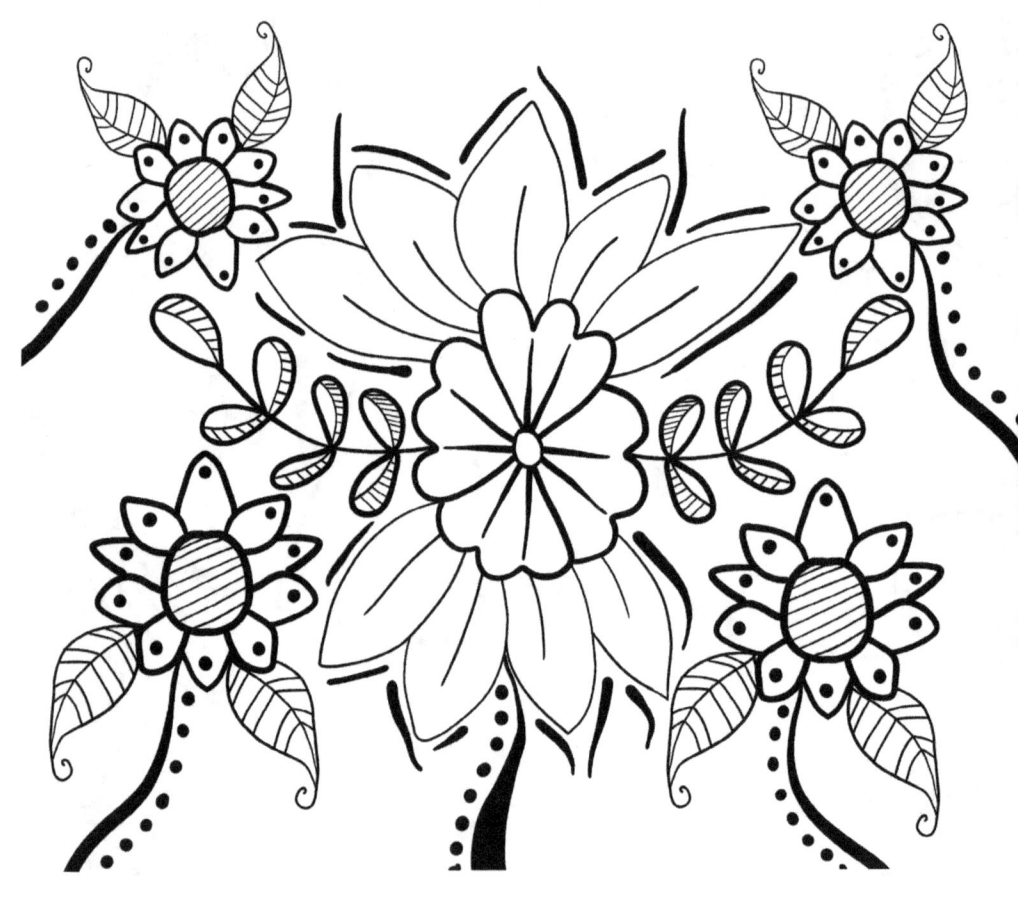

If You're Happy and You Know It, It's Your Meds

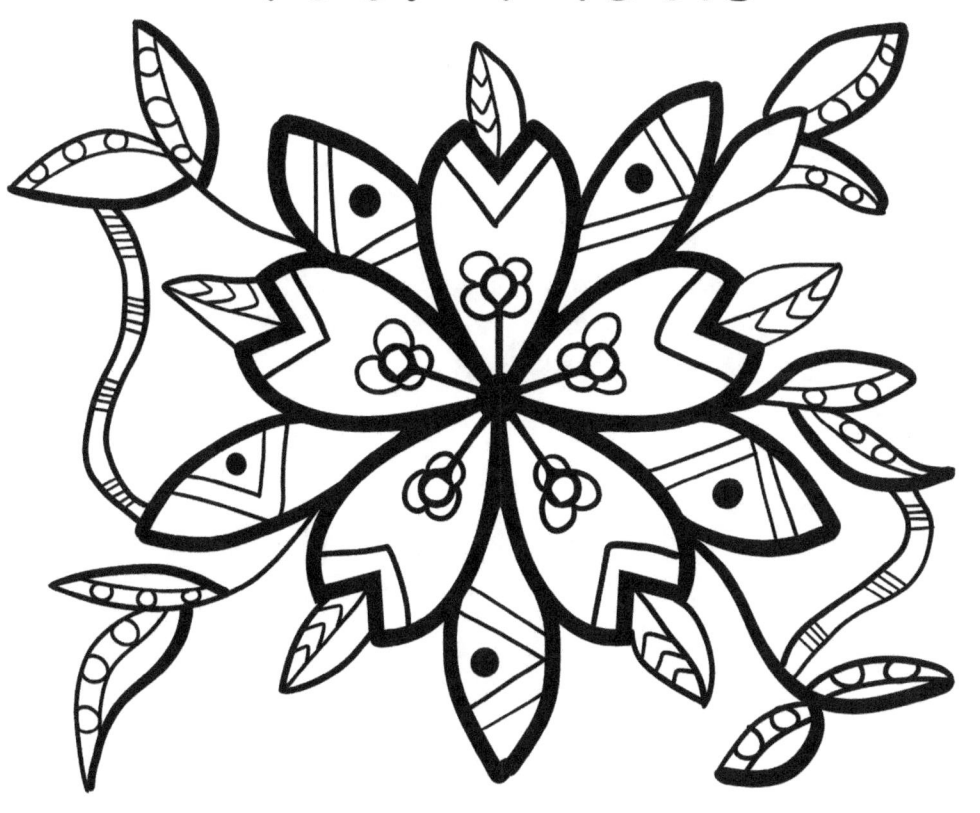